THE RAY PEAT
SURVIVAL GUIDE

BY JOEY LOTT

www.joeylotthealth.com

Publishing services provided by **Archangel Ink**

ISBN: 1517511941
ISBN-13: 978-1517511944

Table of Contents

Introduction

I've written this book for a very specific person. Let's see if that person is you. Read the following description, and if any of this rings true for you, then you've come to the right place; read on. If not, then move along because this isn't the book for you.

Things haven't been going so well for you healthwise. Maybe you've been in denial about it and you're only just now admitting to yourself that your sleep is terrible, your energy levels suck, and your emotions aren't what you'd like them to be. Or maybe you've known that you've been sick for a long time. Maybe you're hypothyroid. Maybe chronic fatigue. Maybe something else. But you know you feel terrible.

Whether you were in denial or not, you've been trying various ways to help yourself feel better for a while. I mean, you could be the exception, but it's extremely rare that someone is interested in Ray Peat's ideas unless they have first exhausted all other "reasonable" alternatives. Most likely you've tried various diets. You may have tried paleo, low carb, zero carb, vegan, low fat, low calorie, sugar free, and so on. And whatever may have seemed to work or not, in the end, nothing lived up to the promises or hopes. In fact, if you're like most people who start investigating Ray Peat's ideas, then those other diets ultimately made you feel worse. Now you may have insulin resistance (common on low carb diets), hair loss, loss of sex drive, constipation, edema, cold intolerance, icy hands and feet, worsening hypothyroidism, insomnia, etc.

So now you're grasping at straws, and you came across mention of Ray Peat on the internet. Maybe at first you were terrified to believe that he may be right, but then you started to open your mind a little. Now, either you're experimenting with the ideas or you're considering it.

But you have doubts. You have fears. You want to get it right. You want to get it perfect. Because now you feel so sick that you don't want to risk making things worse.

Oh, and did I mention that probably half or more of you have a history of restrictive eating disorders? Maybe you have admitted this to yourself. Or maybe you haven't. But at least half have a history of fear of food, fear of gaining weight, fear of losing control, fear of getting sick, fear of being dirty or impure, or any of the other fears and anxieties that make up restrictive eating disorders.

If I've gotten pretty close with my description, then I strongly believe that this book can help you. And I know you because I've been there. I struggled with severely restrictive eating disorders for over 20 years. I tried just about every diet you can imagine. I was obsessed with perfection and purity, and I got sicker and sicker over the years until I was genuinely (and rightfully) concerned for my life. It was only after I had exhausted every other alternative that seemed reasonable to me that I finally became open to hearing the ideas of Ray Peat.

And then, I'll tell you what I did, which is the mistake that many people who begin to explore the ideas of Ray Peat make. I tried to do the Peat-inspired diet/lifestyle perfectly. I tried to be pure.

And, guess what? As a result, like so many Peat adherents, I transferred the same old disordered habits to the new Peat-inspired facade. Ironically, this only served to perpetuate the longstanding chronic stress and the misery that were helping to maintain the illness and the unpleasant symptoms that I started with.

Stress and Ray Peat would probably be the first to tell you this is the number one killer. If you can't ditch the stress, then no matter how much gelatin you eat, no matter how much orange juice you drink, no matter how many thyroid pills you pop, and no matter how much red light you shine on yourself, you'll have a hard time recovering fully.

So in this book, my main hope is to share with you what I believe to be the genius of Ray Peat's ideas, while also sparing you from the mistake of turning "Peatarianism" into the next phase of a worsening cycle of sickness and misery. Truly, for the overwhelming majority of people, there is absolutely no need to do it all so "perfectly" and "purely." In fact, learning to let go of some of that compulsion to do it perfectly and purely may go a long way in helping you to feel better. Really. I know that you probably imagine that you are the exception, but the chances are that you are not. Before you commit yourself to a lifetime of nothing but milk, orange juice, and aspirin washed down with Mexican Coca Cola, I suggest that you be willing to explore what I share with you in this book with an open mind.

The Genius

We live in a world that is dominated by corporate interests. The grip of these interests is so far reaching and so deeply rooted that just about everyone, including most "alternative" health researchers, is in that grip, many without even knowing it. The medical industry is in cahoots with the pharmaceutical industry. The pharmaceutical industry is in cahoots with the agricultural industry. The agricultural industry *is* the chemical industry. And the relationship of all of those industries with the military and the government is complex and incestuous.

So it is rare to find someone with truly original and independent ideas. Ray Peat is one such person.

Does that make Ray Peat right? No. Does that make him infallible? No. Does that make his work a single monolith? No.

But Ray Peat has some original ideas, he's a radically independent thinker, and as best I can tell, he's got a good heart. His ideas are theoretically sound, though certainly not beyond refute, and many of his ideas hold up where the rubber meets the road; people benefit by putting those ideas into practice.

There is much good to say about Ray Peat's work. In my view, the primary messages of genius that come from Ray Peat are as follows:

Trust your own experience and your innate capacity to learn, grow, discover, and adapt. Abandon faith in systems that don't care about you particularly those that actively seek to take advantage of you for their own benefit.

The medical/pharmaceutical/agricultural industry is lying to you about many things.

Sugar is not evil. In fact, at worst it is neutral and at best it is therapeutic and a powerful, beneficial energy source.

Polyunsaturated fat in large amounts for most people is likely unhealthy, whereas saturated fat is protective and nourishing.

Thyroid hormones are crucial for a vast array of metabolic functions in the body, and so protecting, healing, and nourishing the thyroid is essential to good health.

Salt (i.e. sodium chloride) is not the evil that we've been told, and it is actually therapeutic.

Increasing estrogen or serotonin may be a very bad idea.

The values of the culture in which we live are often in conflict with the wellbeing of the individual.

Ultimately, even though I know that Peat may view his work differently, my own summation of his message is this: Think for yourself. Yes, Peat espouses very specific views, but the message of his life the message that emanates from his person and his work is to challenge the status quo and think for yourself, basing your views on what is experientially true versus what is theoretically appealing.

Unfortunately (at least from my perspective), the radical genius of Peat's work and life frequently gets distorted to fit into the narrow ideologies of those who learn of him. Instead of hearing the core message to think for yourself, all too many of us have sought to create a new religion or a new morality from Peat's suggestions particularly his dietary suggestions.

The irony of this is great. Peat writes an entire article about what he sees as the brilliance of William Blake, and in that article, he makes it clear that one of the qualities that he most admires in Blake is his originality and his ability to see things as they are without the burden of dogma and doctrine. Peat clearly holds these values dear, and he clearly seeks to live these values in his own life.

Peat is obviously anti-authoritarian, and so it is ironic that many try to turn him into an authority. I have never spoken with Peat, but I suspect that he would reject the role as authority, and, if you truly read his writings, he has never represented himself as such. Instead, he offers opinions and insights based on a

The Cult

The problem with Peat isn't so much Peat as it is his cult following. Within that subculture, there is often an understandable zeal that distorts the genius of Peat into doctrine. Unfortunately, that is what many of us who are looking for answers end up reading and learning.

Peat's writing is not the easiest to read. Partly, this is because he is an intellectual and he writes like one, but this is also because he's not actually offering a how to, step-by-step, one-size-fits-all solution. If you're looking for that, then you'll be disappointed.

The result is often that within the cult of Peat we end up with dumbed down, step-by--step guides for how to follow the perfect Peat lifestyle. Unfortunately, this usually results in an ultrarestrictive dietary regime with a short list of strong supplements. This approach is neither ideal nor even appropriate for the majority of people.

If Peat actually intended a one-size-fits-all approach, then wouldn't he have written a dietary guide? Instead, he offers personal nutritional counseling. Why? Presumably because he understands that the needs of the individual are highly personal. What is needed by one is not precisely what is needed by another. Although he does often make clear his views of sugar, starch, polyunsaturated fats, proteins, and so forth, surely these guidelines are to be seen as guidelines rather than as dogma.

I will briefly sum up the cliché Peat diet as presented by most involved in the cult. At all costs, one is to avoid excess polyunsaturated fat, estrogen, starch, inflammatory amino acids, phosphorus, lactic acid, iron, endotoxin, and serotonin. Meanwhile, one is to get enough noninflammatory protein, sugar, salt, calcium, magnesium, saturated fat, vitamin A, and vitamin E. Therefore, Peat cultists advise eating only milk, orange juice, some potatoes, gelatin, eggs, cheese, coconut oil, raw carrot, and occasional liver and oysters. All should be well-salted. Then, the cultists advise us to supplement with sugar, aspirin, progesterone, and pregnenolone, all washed down with coffee and a Mexican Coke.

This diet may well be the "perfect" and "pure" diet by Peat standards, but it's rigid, it's dogmatic, and the essence of this approach is antithetical to the core message of Peat's work.

The approach advised by many cultists is too rigid for most people, and for those with a history of restrictive eating disorders, this approach is a recipe for disaster.

The good news is that it is entirely possible to take the genius of Peat and incorporate that into a flexible, adaptive, healthy lifestyle that supports healing, health, and happiness. That is what I hope to show you in this book.

The Dietary Guidelines

As I have already hinted, what draws many people to Peat's work and what many people tend to fixate on are Peat's dietary recommendations. What is interesting to me is that although Peat does make general dietary recommendations throughout his writing, I have yet to come across anything he has written that explicitly spells out what he believes to be the perfect and pure diet. As I have suggested earlier, I believe that he has not done this precisely because he understands that the specific needs of the individual are nuanced and variable, so there is no one-size-fits-all approach.

In this section, I'd like to review the general guidelines that Peat proposes. We'll look at

Mexican Coca-Cola (which is made with cane sugar instead of corn syrup).

This is where many Peatarians make the mistake of trying to make a one-size-fits-all diet plan based on a few anecdotal reports. Just because Ray Peat enjoys that diet and seems to do well on that diet does not mean that this is the only diet that will work for all people. Some people do not do well with orange juice or milk. Some people prefer other types of sugar. Some people thrive on more sugar and some people on less. Some people thrive on bananas (which Peat apparently does not favor), while others thrive on apples (which Peat also does not favor). Some people do very well with maple syrup and/or molasses (both of which Peat suggests may be allergenic for some people a statement that many Peatarians have taken to mean that all people should avoid them). Some people do very well on unrefined cane sugar. Others do better with refined cane sugar. Some people do better without cane sugar.

The point being (and this is a point that I will repeat throughout) that there really, truly is no one-size-fits-all approach. However, Peat's views on sugars may open the eyes and minds of many who have been fearful of sugar, and that is a very good thing. Whatever your personal relationship is with sugars of various sorts, it is good to respect that your body will need sugars in varying amounts and of various sorts at different times. It is good to be willing to trust your body's cravings instead of a rigid ideology. If you crave sugar of any sort, then trust the intelligence of your body.

Next, in the Peat cult, many often misrepresent Peat's writings and suggest that Peat is "antistarch." In actuality, this claim is unsupported by the facts. In Peat's writing, he does suggest in several cases that he believes that sugar is preferable to starch for several reasons. For one thing, he claims that starch creates a larger insulin response than sugar, and therefore starch is more likely to be stored as fat instead of being metabolized directly.

However, Peat also acknowledges that starch can be a part of a healthy diet. This is a fact that is borne out by the longstanding cultures that rely upon starch (rice, potato, wheat, corn, etc.) as an essential part of their diet. And while many Peatarians are quick to try to cut out most starch, they overlook the fact that Peat himself speaks highly of potatoes and is on the record as stating that masa (traditionally-prepared corn), white rice, and oats are potentially valuable parts of a diet. So the starch phobia that is rampant among many in the Peat cult is unfounded.

The bottom line is that Peat advocates for eating sugar and/or starch. In the absence of adequate carbohydrates, thyroid and liver function becomes suppressed, among other potential complications (such as insulin resistance). These are often the outcomes of low carbohydrate diets, so Peat's view on this matter isn't actually farfetched.

Peat advocates for always eating carbohydrates (sugar or starch) along with any protein. Protein, eaten alone, will stimulate insulin secretion. In the absence of dietary carbohydrates, the insulin will lower blood sugar and create a response that includes stress hormones, such as adrenaline and cortisol. This can produce undesirable symptoms and produce longer-term imbalances in the body, so eating carbohydrates with protein is a logical practice.

That should cover sugar and starch, but what about fiber? Well, Peat's main objection to most fiber is that it is estrogenic. Much of the fiber from grains (bran), nuts, and seeds is estrogenic. Peat also argues that fiber from these sources and from most vegetables tends to irritate the digestive system and can therefore increase serotonin (which is also a no-no in Peat's view).

However, it is a mistake to characterize Peat's view of fiber as being strictly anti-fiber. In fact, Peat promotes the idea of eating raw carrot regularly. He also advocates for eating potatoes and some fruits. So he is selective in his views on fiber.

The problem with Peat's published views on fiber is that they don't seem to follow a strictly logical path. Although he speaks highly of potatoes because of their quality protein (in his view) content as well as some vitamins and minerals, potatoes otherwise contain starch and fiber, which aren't consistent with his other stated views. Fruit contains fiber, but he doesn't typically have much caution against fruit (well, except for half the types of fruits that are commercially available). And carrots, which he recommends eating raw (though not cooked), contain glucosinolates in substantial quantities substances that suppress thyroid function (and Peat is generally quite sensitive to anything that might suppress thyroid function).

Given this information, I don't think it is advisable to take Peat's views regarding fiber too far. Rather, I suggest that Peat's general cautions against fiber - particularly insoluble fiber, such as that which is found in large amounts in grain bran and various vegetables, legumes, nuts, and seeds - are a welcome counterbalance to the mainstream's (read: agricultural/medical/pharmaceutical/govern mental) push for increased fiber intake.

It turns out that the backstory behind the current bran/fiber craze is not as wholesome as we've been led to believe. In fact, the foundations of the fiber craze are rooted in unsubstantiated hypotheses. In the 1970's, a man named Denis Burkitt formed a hypothesis that dietary fiber accounted for what he saw as an absence of certain diseases among some African populations. Since then, the studies regarding the role of fiber in disease have shown mixed results. There are some very intelligent and detailed critiques of the fiber hypothesis that are well beyond the scope of this book. However, suffice it to say that the jury is still out in regard to the fiber hypothesis, and there is good evidence to support that in many cases, such as irritable bowel syndrome or Crohn's disease, dietary fiber, particularly insoluble fiber, can be a big problem.

So Peat's views on fiber, like his views on many things, may help to offer some balance. If you truly enjoy eating bran, beans, and broccoli in excess, and if you thrive on that, then by all means listen to the intelligence of your body. But if you are one of the many people who eat large amounts of insoluble fiber because you've been convinced to do so for "health" reasons, then you may find Peat's views to be refreshing. (And, by the way, John Harvey Kellogg, the famous co-inventor of corn flakes, ran a sanitarium in Michigan where he prescribed diets high in insoluble fiber as a means to treat constipation. However, he found that the insoluble fiber eventually bound people up! So he began to add mineral oil to the food, and he prescribed daily enemas. Be cautious of the claims that large amounts of insoluble fiber are necessary for a healthy colon. In fact, it would seem that any laxative effects are often short term, eventually leading to bowel irritation and injury.)

In summary:

• Peat recommends eating substantial carbohydrates, favoring sugar to starch, but by no means suggesting that starch is inherently problematic for all people. If you enjoy, crave, or desire carbohydrates, then please honor the intelligence of your body, and eat!

• Peat suggests that sugar in particular, in the absence of excess polyunsaturated fat, may be therapeutic in many cases, including cases of insulin resistance, hyperglycemia, and diabetes. Peat suggests that much, or perhaps even all, of the cautions against sugar may be unfounded and even wrong.

• Peat recommends eating carbohydrates with protein any time protein is eaten to avoid low blood sugar and a stress response.

• Peat suggests that most insoluble fiber is problematic, either because it is estrogenic or because it irritates the intestines, possibly producing excess serotonin.

• Although many Peatarians try to turn this advice into a rigid dogma that allows for only milk and orange juice, the truth is that Peat's guidelines and recommendations in regard to carbohydrates allow a great deal of flexibility. The bottom line is to allow yourself to eat what you desire without placing artificial restrictions on yourself, and adjust if necessary based on biofeedback. If you crave sugar in any form, then trust that instinct, and eat what you crave. If you crave starch, then trust that instinct.

Fat

Peat's views on fat are rather emphatic and straightforward. He argues repeatedly that polyunsaturated fats of all kinds are potentially harmful and should be avoided to whatever extent possible. He also says that while the body is capable of producing fats from carbohydrates, it is sensible to eat some dietary saturated fat. Peat tends to speak highly of coconut oil for this purpose, though he is also in favor of butter fat, which is also highly saturated.

Peat's argument for why unsaturated fats, and polyunsaturated fats specifically, are problematic is that they cause inflammation, slow mitochondrial energy production, suppress thyroid function, inhibit detoxification, and suppress immunity.

He argues that the industrial (agricultural/pharmaceutical/governmental/etc.) push of polyunsaturated fats is rooted in profits rather than sound research and a genuine interest in the health and wellbeing of the population. He cites numerous studies that demonstrate the effects that he attributes to polyunsaturated fat.

Truthfully, Peat seems to turn polyunsaturated fat into as near as a demon as possible. And, to be honest, in the right context he makes a very strong argument. The only context I see in which his argument doesn't hold up is in the traditional diets of people living in extreme latitudes. People like the Inuit traditionally ate diets composed mostly of large amounts of polyunsaturated fats, as are found in the fish, seals, and whales that they hunted. And, all things considered, it would seem that these people have fared quite well, especially considering the extremely inhospitable environments in which they live. However, it is notable that their diets include extremely low amounts of carbohydrates, instead relying largely on fat for their energy. Plus, given the extremely cold environment, it is reasonable to assume that the people in that environment would fare better with dietary polyunsaturated fat than people living in temperate or tropical environments.

Frankly, I think that Peat's arguments against polyunsaturated fat are so good that I expect that it is reasonable for most people to experiment with reducing polyunsaturated fat intake and favoring saturated fat instead. For most people, this is not difficult since most people typically enjoy butter to canola oil. In fact, many people find that after taking a break from polyunsaturated fat staples, such as nuts, seeds, polyunsaturated vegetable oils, and the like, they have no appetite for those things.

Some people, however, take this to an unnecessary extreme. They try to eliminate very nearly all polyunsaturated fat from their diet without regard for the implications. While many people may benefit greatly by reducing dietary polyunsaturated fat, it is clear to me that this has to be done in a healthy, sustainable, and enjoyable way. Normally, reducing polyunsaturated fat isn't difficult because most people usually prefer butter to canola oil and beef fat to chicken fat. And normally, if a person is eating enough variety of palatable, enjoyable foods, then there is little craving for large amounts of nuts or seeds. But what can happen with overzealous elimination of polyunsaturated fat is that some people can inadvertently reduce their caloric intake or their protein intake, which can have harmful health effects in many cases. Furthermore, if you eliminate polyunsaturated fat without regard for the genuine cravings of the body, then you may inadvertently deprive your body of needed nutrition.

So while I agree that reducing polyunsaturated fat is likely to be helpful for many, if not most people, I believe that there is a helpful way to approach this and an unhelpful way to approach this. To begin with, I strongly suggest that you listen to your body. If your body genuinely craves polyunsaturated fat, then do not reject that just because Ray Peat doesn't like polyunsaturated fat, no matter how good his arguments are. Secondly, replace polyunsaturated fats with equal calories that are palatable and enjoyable to you. If you approach this transition with too much zeal, then you may eliminate polyunsaturated fat without replacing it with adequate energy. It is important that the food that you eat is enjoyable, palatable, and fulfilling to you in order to make the dietary practices truly sustainable for you.

I also encourage you to avoid the temptation to try to eliminate all polyunsaturated fats. For one thing, it's an impossibility, since just about any fat of any sort contains some polyunsaturated fat. Even coconut oil, which is highly saturated, contains some polyunsaturated fat. Instead, simply become aware of the sources of large amounts of polyunsaturated fats, and then replace those fats with a combination of carbohydrates, protein, and saturated fat to whatever extent is enjoyable and sustainable for you.

Some of the common sources of large amounts of polyunsaturated fat include all non-tropical vegetable oils (i.e. soy, corn, canola, safflower, sunflower, sesame, flax, etc.), nuts (i.e. almonds, walnuts, Brazil nuts, etc.), seeds, poultry fat, and pork fat.

Common sources of saturated fat include butter, suet, and coconut oil. Ray Peat seems to have a particularly favorable opinion of coconut oil. If you happen to like coconut oil, then using more coconut oil in your cooking is probably easy. However, even those of us who once-upon-a-time enjoyed coconut oil tend to develop a distaste for it. (Reportedly, refined coconut oil is largely tasteless, which works well for many people.) Butter, on the other hand, tends to be quite enjoyable to most people most of the time.

So does this mean that you should never eat Brazil nuts, chicken, or bacon ever again? No. It does not.

If you crave nuts, seeds, poultry fat, or pork fat, then eat them to whatever extent you genuinely crave them. However, you may find that simply being cognizant of polyunsaturated fats and experimenting with reducing them may reveal some benefits for you. Also, many people find that the fat from poultry or pork doesn't actually agree with them. Skinless chicken (particularly a low fat cut, such as the breast), however, is relatively low in polyunsaturated fat, so it is not necessary to give up poultry and pork completely. Peat himself reportedly eats bacon. He fries it, discards the fat, and then cooks it again in coconut oil.

I'm not suggesting that you should become neurotic at all about polyunsaturated fat. Rather, I am sharing with you the Peat perspective and hopefully tempering that with the recommendation that you experiment and be willing to trust in your body both in the cravings and in the biofeedback (i.e. how you feel after eating various foods).

Protein

Ray Peat is a fan of protein primarily because he views protein as being pro-thyroid in nature. Though he doesn't advocate for a high protein diet, he does suggest that adequate protein requirements for most people are likely higher than the governmental recommendations of less than 50 grams per day. He has written that he personally doesn't feel very good eating less than 100 grams per day, and he typically eats closer to 150 grams per day.

However, Peat offers some caveats to this. He most certainly does not advocate for a protein free-for-all. He claims that with the exception of potatoes, the only other quality proteins are from animal foods, and he warns against eating too much protein that is high in inflammatory amino acids, such as tryptophan, cysteine, and methionine. Also, while adequate protein is important, Peat doesn't suggest that more than enough is better.

Ray Peat often speaks (or writes) favorably about dairy sources of protein. Cheese, in particular, Peat says is best because it is very low in tryptophan. Peat is also quite fond of gelatin, which is deficient in tryptophan (inflammatory) and an exceedingly good source of glycine (antiinflammatory). Although he does advocate for the judicious inclusion of muscle meat and organ meat in the diet, he cautions that these meats are high in inflammatory amino acids, and he recommends eating them with gelatin. He makes a good point, which is that muscle meat and organ meat represent only part of the whole animal. Traditionally, the entire animal would be eaten, which includes a fairly massive amount of collagen (gelatin). He also speaks favorably of eggs as a protein source since the protein quality is high with a balanced amino acid profile, and eggs are very nutrient dense (mostly in the yolks). He does caution against eating too many eggs in the long run because of the polyunsaturated fat content, though.

So really, there's not a great deal to get neurotic about when it comes to Peat's protein views, and yet, many of us have found ways to become neurotic about protein, using Peat's views as an excuse. For one thing, many people eschew muscle meat altogether because it is inflammatory on its own. This is, of course, simply inverting the mistake that we began with by eating only muscle meat. While I have heard reports from some who are eating 150 grams of gelatin a day along with dairy or eggs, this seems just as silly as eating nothing but steaks. Then some people try to force themselves to eat more protein than they actually want or need simply because Peat is on record as saying that he eats 150 grams of protein per day on average.

What a lot of people miss is that most foods have some protein. Even if the quality of the protein isn't the greatest (as in most fruits, vegetables, or starches), the combination with other foods tends to create a more or less balanced protein. So if you drink a pint of orange juice (4 grams of protein) with an egg (6 grams of protein), an ounce of cheddar cheese (7 grams of protein), and a potato (4 grams of protein), then that's 21 grams of protein. And even if the protein in the orange juice isn't the greatest quality, when combined with the other protein, it balances out.

So it isn't necessary to eat 150 grams of gelatin or drink a gallon of milk every day to meet your protein requirement.

Furthermore, everybody's protein requirements are different, and they change over time. Just because Ray Peat need 100150 grams a day doesn't mean that you do, but if you find that you aren't feeling so great and you typically eat less than, say, 70 grams of protein a day, then you may want to experiment with ways to increase your protein intake in enjoyable and palatable ways. See if that helps you to feel better.

Don't be afraid of eating what you enjoy eating, either. Not everyone wants to eat a lot of cheese. And not everyone fares well on a diet with lots of dairy as the primary protein source. If you enjoy eating steaks, then eat steaks. If you don't like gelatin, then don't eat it just because you think you should. But then again, be willing to branch out and try new things. Again, let your cravings and biofeedback be your guide.

Minerals

The oversimplified summary of Ray Peat's views on minerals is as follows: Calcium, sodium, and magnesium are good. Phosphorus, iron, and iodine in excess are bad. Otherwise, he doesn't typically express much one way or the other about minerals apart from stating that a diet should include an adequate supply of minerals, including trace minerals.

Calcium and phosphorus oppose one another, and so Peat's view is that the most important consideration in regard to these two minerals is the ratio. He normally suggests that it is ideal to consume more calcium than phosphorus.

According to Peat, calcium is beneficial because it reduces the activity of both the parathyroid and the pituitary, both of which he says oppose the activity of the thyroid. In other words, when parathyroid and pituitary activity are high, thyroid activity is suppressed. Since Peat views thyroid activity as being essential to good health, he generally doesn't hold a positive opinion of anything that opposes thyroid function, so calcium's action of reducing parathyroid and pituitary activity is a good thing in his view.

On the other hand, according to Peat, excessive, unopposed phosphorus leads to a whole lot of unpleasant symptoms ranging from fatigue to cancer to osteoporosis. To be clear, he does not advocate for trying to achieve an extreme reduction in dietary phosphorus. Rather, he suggests that emphasizing foods that have a high calcium to phosphorus ratio may be beneficial.

According to Peat, foods that have a high phosphorus to calcium ratio (not good) include muscle meat, fish, beans, and whole grains. Foods with a high calcium to phosphorus ratio (good) include milk and cheese. He also mentions leafy greens in this category, though most of the time he holds aboveground plants (not including fruits) in low regard.

Of course, it is possible to take this to an extreme and try to exclude all foods that are high in phosphorus and low in calcium, but this is unnecessary and also not what Peat is advocating. Rather, Peat simply advocates for having awareness of the overall dietary phosphorus to calcium ratio, and he suggests that you are likely to feel better if you eat more calcium than phosphorus overall. Natural dietary sources of calcium include bone broth and eggshell flour, if you feel that you need supplemental calcium.

Sodium is a mineral that is much maligned in the mainstream. It is blamed for high blood pressure and other maladies. However, Peat suggests that much of these opinions may be unfounded. In fact, Peat believes that sodium, particularly sodium chloride (table salt, sea salt, or rock salt), has many therapeutic uses, including reducing inflammation, inducing thermogenesis, increasing carbon dioxide levels, improving sleep, and more. He also suggests that sodium helps with magnesium retention. So overall, Peat suggests that the inclusion of adequate dietary salt can be health-promoting.

Peat claims that like calcium, a deficiency in magnesium can also cause parathyroid stimulation, which, in turn, opposes thyroid activity. Furthermore, he points out that magnesium is needed to balance and keep in check the activity of calcium in the body. Because of this, Peat advises that maintaining magnesium levels is important. As far as I can tell, the only sources of magnesium that he promotes are coffee, cacao/chocolate, and Epsom salt baths. While Peat is very big on coffee, I'm not sure that he's right on this one. Other than espresso, other types of coffee contain relatively small amounts of magnesium with large amounts of phytic acid that binds to the magnesium and other minerals in the digestive tract.

Peat warns against excessive iodine supplementation as is popular in certain circles of people following the advice of doctors, such as David Brownstein, who promote supplementation with extremely large doses. Peat has expressed the view that large amounts of iodine are likely to suppress the thyroid rather than heal it.

Finally, we get to iron, which is the mineral devil in Peat's writings. He does not have a favorable opinion of iron, which is a heavy metal that oxidizes easily. Peat claims that excess iron plays a role in cancer, heart disease, Parkinson's disease, ALS, Alzheimer's, and more. Peat even claims that while iron deficiency can and does exist, it is much rarer than we imagine, and that it is rarely the cause of anemia. (He says that iron may stimulate red blood cell formation, but he also argues that arsenic or radiation will stimulate red blood cell formation. Might it be just as sensible to argue that cases of anemia are due to arsenic deficiency?)

Since iron accumulates, Peat advises against eating too much. He advocates for drinking coffee with meals that include iron-containing foods, such as red meat or eggs, because he says that coffee inhibits iron absorption.

Vitamins

Peat speaks primarily of three officially recognized vitamins and caffeine, which he claims should be considered a vitamin. He seems to feel that Vitamin A, Vitamin D, and Vitamin E all have a broad range of therapeutic value.

Vitamin A, according to Peat, opposes estrogen and is therefore important. He suggests that too little Vitamin A can cause problems, and as such, he recommends eating eggs and occasional liver. However, he cautions that because Vitamin A is unsaturated, it may suppress thyroid function in excess.

When Peat speaks of Vitamin A, he is only speaking of retinoids, which are the active form found in animal foods. Other compounds, such as carotenoids that are found in plant foods, are not always successfully converted to the active form in humans, so the active form is the only sure way to get dietary Vitamin A. In addition, Peat is not a fan of carotenoids, because he views them as potentially dangerous polyunsaturated fatty acids. (Frankly, I am not convinced of this. I think this claim may be a bit over the top, but it's also possible that he's right.)

As I mentioned, Peat cites eggs and liver as good sources of Vitamin A. However, butter is actually a superior source to eggs, and cheese is similar to eggs. Peat is right about liver, though, which is one of the richest food sources of Vitamin A. Because of the nutritional density of liver, Peat advises eating a serving of liver once every week or two and no more often.

Peat also mentions Vitamin D on occasion. Since he thinks favorably of calcium, it is not surprising that he suggests that sufficient Vitamin D is also important (Vitamin D helps with calcium absorption). He also suggests that Vitamin D helps to retain both calcium and magnesium. He has advised some people to supplement with Vitamin D when they do not get enough sunlight (since Vitamin D is normally produced on the skin when exposed to sunlight).

However, he also cautions that excessive Vitamin D can be estrogenic. Interestingly, he cites a study that indicates that (at least in rats) the effects of a Vitamin D deficiency may be offset by eating sugar in place of starch.

Vitamin E is one of Ray Peat's darlings, though interestingly, he rarely advocates for supplementing with it. He's on the record as saying that much of the present day Vitamin E supplements are of inferior quality. In any case, Peat has written that Vitamin E is anti-inflammatory, and it opposes estrogen. Plus, Vitamin E can ameliorate the negative effects of polyunsaturated fats. Rumor has it that Peat has advised some people to supplement with Vitamin E before eating a large amount of polyunsaturated fat, though I cannot substantiate this claim. The only problem is, as I have already stated, Peat doesn't seem to think there are any quality Vitamin E supplements on the market today.

Finally, Peat argues that caffeine is "vitamin-like." He attributes a long list of benefits to caffeine, including liver protection, hormonal balance, cancer protection, energy efficiency, nerve protection, and more. Peat's favorite caffeine source is coffee, which we'll cover in more depth in the next section.

Coffee

Coffee is a Ray Peat favorite. Although the mainstream view of coffee is that it is a vice to be reduced or eliminated whenever possible, Peat defends coffee as a superfood par excellence.

Coffee is Peat's favorite source of caffeine, to begin with, and, as I mentioned in the previous section, Peat views caffeine as a vitamin-like substance. He lists many potential benefits to caffeine, including those that I listed in the preceding section.

Peat says that the negative effects that are normally attributed to caffeine and coffee are actually the result of improved sugar metabolism the result being possible hypoglycemia, which produces a stress response. So Peat's solution? Sugar. Peat claims that simply adding sugar (or starch as in drinking coffee with a meal or with cake or something like that) will completely resolve the potential problems. In other words, Peat is saying that simply adding sufficient sugar to your coffee should completely eliminate any jittery feelings.

Apart from the benefits of caffeine, Peat likes coffee for other reasons. Perhaps the reason that he cites most often is that coffee reportedly can inhibit the absorption of iron, which is why he recommends drinking coffee with any iron-rich food.

Peat also says that coffee can block phosphorus. You may recall that according to Peat, phosphorus has negative effects if unchecked. So coffee's ability to block phosphorus is yet another benefit.

Peat claims that coffee protects the thyroid from cancer, removes heavy metals, and is a good source of magnesium and Vitamin B1. (Though, to be honest, I believe that to get significant quantities of magnesium from coffee, even in theory, you need to drink espresso.)

Peat must drink a lot of coffee. I have never seen reports of just how much, but he certainly doesn't seem to caution against drinking too much! Of course, everyone is different. Some people enjoy coffee. Some don't. Some do well with coffee. Some don't. So you have to use your own good judgment to determine what is right for you.

Supplements

Peat is on record as advocating for the use of several supplements under some conditions. Namely, he suggests that aspirin, thyroid hormone, pregnenolone, and progesterone may be helpful for some people some of the time.

Peat likes aspirin, because it opposes estrogen and polyunsaturated fatty acids. He says that in an ideal world, none of us would have been exposed to excess polyunsaturated fat (which he says replaces natural fatty acids in the body) or excess estrogen. However, given the situation, Peat believes that aspirin is as near a panacea as possible.

He refutes the claim that aspirin causes stomach ulcers, saying that the studies that showed stomach ulcer formation were giving the equivalent of 10 to 100 aspirin tablets at once under conditions that were designed to form ulcers. He says that to the contrary, aspirin can protect against ulcers when used appropriately.

Of course, your mileage may vary. Some people seem to tolerate aspirin quite well while others do not. Supplementing with aspirin may be ill-advised for some people.

I must say that I don't have any personal desire to supplement with aspirin. However, Peat's views opened my eyes to my biases. I saw aspirin as a drug with the sole purpose of relieving pain. I put aspirin into a category separate from things that I considered to be nutritional supplements things like vitamins or minerals. But it was curious to notice that the classification on my part was quite arbitrary. It's interesting for me to notice that I am not particularly hesitant to recommend supplementing with Vitamin D, for example, but I have hesitation recommending supplemental aspirin or hormones (interestingly, of course, Vitamin D actually is a hormone!), such as pregnenolone or progesterone. So again, I encourage you to have an open mind and explore the biases that you may have surrounding these issues.

Peat speaks highly of supplemental thyroid hormone on more than one occasion. He often refers to a product called Cytomel (or

Cynomel) that contains only T3 hormone, which is the "active" thyroid hormone. I haven't seen him make much mention of desiccated thyroid glandular, though the few offhand references he has included in his writing sound favorable. What is clear from his writing is that he does not believe that synthetic T4 supplements are a good idea.

Although supplemental thyroid does seem to help a lot of people, I wonder if it is a good first approach. Often times, Peatarians resort to supplemental thyroid as a first approach before considering factors like whether or not they are eating enough calories.

Peat also likes supplemental pregnenolone. He claims that it is totally nontoxic, and he says that in those with adequate pregnenolone levels, utilizing supplemental pregnenolone will have no effect. However, for those with low pregnenolone levels, Peat claims that supplementing even with large amounts (he is rumored to have used 3 grams a day for a time) has no unpleasant side effects.

Some anecdotal reports from self--proclaimed Peatarians suggest that supplemental pregnenolone, even in moderate doses, may cause unpleasant side effects, including aggression and insomnia. On the other hand, most note only positive or neutral effects.

Finally, Peat is a fan of supplemental progesterone. This hormone, he cautions, is not a male hormone (meaning that men naturally produce very small amounts of the hormone), and therefore, it is generally not appropriate for men to supplement with it. (He does note that there may be exceptions. Some men do find that supplementing with progesterone can be helpful in some cases.) Peat likes progesterone because it opposes the effects of estrogen. For women, he claims that supplemental progesterone between ovulation and menstruation can alleviate the symptoms of PMS. He also makes recommendations for supplementation with progesterone for perimenopausal and postmenopausal women.

In summary, I will add my own commentary. Although Peat makes good arguments for supplemental aspirin, pregnenolone, and progesterone under certain circumstances, I believe that it is a mistake to resort to supplementing with these substances as a first line of approach. I see many self-professed Peatarians supplementing with these substances before giving adequate attention to eating enough food or other lifestyle considerations (as are discussed later in this book).

Putting Diet in Context

Peat's dietary and supplemental recommendations are insightful and helpful antidotes to the biased information we receive through mainstream channels. Don't get me wrong; I'm not saying that Peat isn't biased. I'm just suggesting that at least Peat's biases are counter to much of what we normally hear, and he provides as much, if not more evidence to back his claims as anything else we might hear. In fact, he does a pretty good job of steering clear of being guilty of rationalism, which I cannot say is true for so much of what we hear coming from other channels.

So I have a great appreciation for Peat's views and his willingness to publish his views, but that doesn't mean that I think that he's right in all cases.

I find that it's helpful to put all of the dietary recommendations into perspective. When we forget the context, it is easy to get carried away and overzealous with any ideas.

Let's look at a specific health concern insulin resistance. In the mainstream, we are told that insulin resistance is caused by a diet consisting of too much sugar and saturated fat, but if that was true, then surely insulin resistance and diabetes would have devastated large numbers of traditional people who relied either on large amounts of sugars (such as Amazonian cultures eating sugar cane and tropical fruits) or large amounts of saturated fats.

Peat, on the other hand, blames insulin resistance on a variety of factors, not the least of which is high dietary intake of polyunsaturated fats. But then wouldn't insulin resistance and diabetes have ravaged traditional people, such as the Inuit, whose diets included significant polyunsaturated fat?

In its own context, it is possible for just about any dietary philosophy to seem to be the one true answer to all health problems. Raw veganism, paleo, low fat, grain free, low carbohydrate, and so on, all provide convincing arguments within an isolated context, but when you take a look at the bigger picture, none of these philosophies have a monopoly on truth.

The reality seems to be that humans have survived and thrived on a wide variety of diets over long periods of time. It seems likely that humans have fared well enough on diets that include gluten, grain, unrefined grain, refined grain, high polyunsaturated fat (although this may be a rare and extreme exception limited to high latitude regions), high saturated fat, low fat, nightshades, no nightshades, lots of fruit, lots of vegetables, raw, cooked, high calorie, low calorie, high carbohydrates, low carbohydrates, and on and on.

Presently, as you read this, there are people who are thriving on a variety of diets some moderate and some extreme. I have to say, however, that it is my observation that those who thrive tend to do so on a more moderate (i.e. unrestrictive) diet rather than on an extreme (i.e. restrictive) diet.

So while Peat has some really valuable insights, I believe that for the overwhelming majority of people, it is a huge mistake to try to convert to pure and perfect Peatarianism as a desperate attempt to feel well. This is not only unlikely to be necessary (or possible) for most people, it is actually likely to be harmful on several levels. For one thing, it is likely to perpetuate the emotional stress and the habitual stress patterns of restrictive, disordered eating and food/health anxiety. For another thing, the restrictive nature of what most people imagine must be the pure and perfect Peat-inspired diet is likely to be too much liquid and not enough calories for the typical hypometabolic person.

So here's what I suggest: use what you learn through Peat's ideas to challenge yourself to let go of everything you think you know. Peat's ideas are often so radically opposed to everything that you thought you knew that it is the perfect opportunity to realize that you never will know all the answers and that no one else knows either.

Then, be inspired by the core of Peat's message. **Think for yourself**. Listen to your own biofeedback. If you crave something, then eat it no matter how much someone else says that thing is bad for you. If you don't want something, then don't eat it no matter how much someone else says that thing is supposedly so healthy for you.

And then adapt and adjust as necessary. If something doesn't seem to sit well with you, then be willing to change something. Be willing to keep adjusting. What you wanted yesterday and what worked yesterday may or may not be the right thing today. And similarly, what did not work yesterday may or may not work today. Trust your body's cravings.

Does that mean that you should totally disregard Peat's views or anyone else's views? No. Of course not. They may be helpful in some regard. For example, if Peat's views on sugar give you permission to explore your desire for sugar, then great. Or if his views on coffee allow you to give yourself permission to drink coffee if you actually want it, then great.

But don't eat sugar and drink coffee if you don't actually want to or if they don't make you feel good just because Peat said so. At the same time, don't assume that just because sugar or coffee or anything else doesn't work for you that it will necessarily always be that way. Trust in the natural intelligence of your body to heal, to adjust, and to signal you with its needs that change from one moment to the next.

The Importance of Lifestyle Factors

The unfortunate thing about Ray Peat's views is that they are often viewed in a very narrow context as if the only or most important things you could do for your health are to drink lots of milk, orange juice, and coffee, and to possibly supplement with aspirin. This is, in my view, a misunderstanding. I believe it is important to view the larger context in which Peat's specific dietary suggestions may be helpful. What follows in this section is Peat's lifestyle recommendations with my additions to round it out.

Really, the foundation of Peat's health outlook seems to be the reduction of stress. In fact, all of Peat's dietary recommendations are about reducing stress. You'll remember that the purpose of eating carbohydrates, adding salt, providing adequate anti-inflammatory protein, and reducing polyunsaturated fat is fundamentally about reducing stress responses.

So it should come as no surprise that the lifestyle context for the dietary recommendations is also all about reducing stress. Peat specifically talks about the importance of light and carbon dioxide in this regard.

Peat's theory is that darkness and blue light are inherently stressful for humans, while red light is de-stressing, so Peat recommends adequate sunlight and supplemental red light (meaning light that is skewed more toward the red end of the spectrum). Of course, some Peatarians take this advice too far and shine heat lamps on themselves at night as they try to sleep. This is likely unnecessary and will probably just upset your spouse, but Peat's general recommendation to get sunlight and to give preference to red light (as in incandescent) instead of blue light (as in fluorescent) when using supplemental lighting is sensible.

Peat views carbon dioxide as an essential nutrient in the human organism. Many of his recommendations, such as the preference for sugar over starch, are based on what will either spare carbon dioxide or produce carbon dioxide in the body. He often writes of the benefits of high altitudes, including a greater carbon dioxide to oxygen level in the air. Peat also recommends rebreathing into a paper bag in times of acute need in order to increase carbon dioxide levels.

Although I have never found a reference to Peat actually endorsing the Buteyko method, he does seem to at least have some respect for it. The Buteyko method is founded upon the theory that reduced breathing volume results in an increase in carbon dioxide retention and a whole host of health benefits. (As a side note, I personally have found benefit from the Buteyko method, particularly practicing with the Frolov device or the less expensive American knockoff, the BreathSlim device.)

Although Peat doesn't explicitly speak of the importance of getting enough quality sleep, he does seem to implicitly acknowledge the importance of quality sleep when he writes about using gelatin and salt to induce and improve sleep and when he writes about the potential harm of supplemental melatonin. Adequate, quality sleep is important for healthy, natural hormone balance. And, of course, adequate, quality sleep is normally a tall order for people in a hypometabolic state. So while improving the metabolic rate is likely to improve sleep quality, I also think that there's a sort of chicken and egg scenario happening; improving sleep can improve metabolism and improving metabolism can improve sleep.

There are other factors involved in stress reduction that I rarely, if ever, see Peat mention. These seem significant enough to me that I will make mention of them here.

With all the emphasis that Peat tends to place on what to eat (or not eat), he rarely says anything of how much to eat. In my research, it does seem that there is a strong connection between undereating and lowered metabolic rate. Peat does at least address this very cursorily in several of his articles when he mentions that calorie restriction in humans tends to reduce metabolic rate, and he does often make it clear that he views hypometabolism as problematic.

As I have mentioned several times throughout the book, I have noticed that many people trying to follow the "perfect" Peat-inspired diet can end up with a caloric deficit. That is because they restrict their diet to a small number of foods, many of them liquid, and frankly, not always terribly palatable. While milk and orange juice are both quite enjoyable at times, it can be difficult to maintain a high enough caloric intake on those foods alone in the long run. And if you are not eating enough calories, then you are more likely to produce a stress response than if you are eating enough calories. So, there is a balance to be struck between keeping in mind some of the principles that Peat espouses and eating what you enjoy. When in doubt, just eat what you enjoy! I find that those who are recovering from restrictive eating often need to let go of all the restrictions and just eat according to appetite even if that means eating fried chicken and corn chips all cooked in canola oil. Eat enough, and make choices based on appetite/desire rather than ideology. This normally will lead you in the right direction. And Peat's views can be liberating in this respect, opening the doors to sugar, starch, saturated fat, salt, coffee, chocolate, and other foods that your ideology may have denied you in the past.

Peat also rarely, if ever, makes mention of the value of stress relief techniques or programs. Instead, he tends to focus on making changes in diet or supplementation as a way to improve the felt emotional experience, but there is plenty of evidence that suggests that the other way around works as well. In other words, effective practices for reducing or releasing stress by way of changes in behavior or meditation or the like can provoke changes in the physiology that support a more stress-free experience of life in the longer term. I have found this to be true, personally. In fact, for those of us who have experienced restrictive eating patterns, with all the anxiety that that entails, I believe a good stress release program is extremely helpful, if not essential.

Finally, I will add that it is important to let go and enjoy life. To his credit, Peat also says as much. He views curiosity and play as essential ingredients for health.

Putting This Into Practice

Ray Peat is fundamentally antiauthoritarian and antiestablishment, so it is perverse that some take his views and try to make it into a religion of sorts. Also, it is a mistake to try to take his general ideas and apply them specifically to all cases.

So how can you take all of this information and put in into practice in a healthy, adaptive way?

My recommendation is this: See that Peat's views are contextual. Understand that he does not have a monopoly on truth. Furthermore, since his work is not a monolith, know that he may be right about some things and wrong about other things. Or, more likely, right about some things some of the time and wrong about some things some of the time.

Listen to your own body. Use anything and everything, including Peat's views, to give yourself permission to ditch the dogma and doctrine. Be willing to experiment. And trust your biofeedback. If you are hungry, then eat. If you are tired, then sleep. If you crave ice cream, then eat ice cream. If you crave potatoes, then eat potatoes. If you crave bacon, then eat bacon fried in coconut oil or not! And then pay attention to how you feel. I'm not suggesting that you become a hypochondriac, worrying about every minor fluctuation in experience, but just trust how you feel as a guidepost. If eating bacon consistently makes you feel terrible, then maybe lay off the bacon.

Steer clear of absolutism. Just because bacon doesn't agree with you once or maybe even for a month, don't restrict bacon for the rest of your life if you find that you crave it. Understand that things change. And likely, as your metabolism improves, you'll have fewer sensitivities.

Also understand that everything doesn't have to be an instant fix. Some things take time. It took you a while to get to the point where you are now, so it might take a few days, weeks, months, or even years to get back to feeling 100%. Have patience. I know that's hard. Really, I do. I know from personal experience the temptation to jump ship and try the next dramatic and extreme fad approach to healing.

Eat enough. Rest enough. Eat some more. Keep eating. Keep resting. Get some sun. Laugh. Smile. Breathe easily and gently. And ditch the stress. Oh, and eat. Did I mention eat?

Please don't turn Peat's views into a religion. Remember that plenty of people are healthy eating in a variety of ways. There is no one true way. There is only what works for you. Peat has some good insights. Chief among them, in my opinion, is that excess polyunsaturated fat is potentially harmful in many cases. His views on salt, adequate quality protein, and a balanced amino acid profile also seem to make good sense. And his view regarding carbohydrates can be liberating if you simply allow yourself to eat again instead of debating whether you should be eating only starch or only sugar. Just eat. Eat what you enjoy. Eat enough.

And let go. Life is better when letting go.

Get My Future Books FREE

If you enjoyed this book (Hey, if you made it this far it couldn't have been that bad), you'll probably enjoy many of my other books about health and wellness. And you can get all my new releases in health and wellness for free by signing up for my mailing list at www.joeylotthealth.com. It's simple, it's free, and it's totally honest and legitimate. Nothing scammy or spammy or anything else like that (i.e. I won't be trying to sell you The 7 Dirty Underground Top Secret Weird Tricks for Rock Hard Abs or Young Living Oils). It's just about free books for those who appreciate my work, because I appreciate YOU. Simple as that.

Connect With Me

I welcome your questions, comments, and feedback of any kind. Please feel free to email me at joeylott@gmail.com. I am now receiving so many emails that I cannot always reply to every email. I do read them all, and I do my best to reply to as many as possible. For the benefit of others, I may choose to publish my response to your email on my blog or in book format. I will maintain your privacy and anonymity if I choose to publish my response.

One Small Favor

My sincere goal in writing is to share something that may be of value to you. And I endeavor to do so while keeping the costs low for readers. The success of my books and my ability to reach other readers who may benefit from my books depends in large part on having lots of thoughtful, honest reviews written about my work. You would do me a great favor if you would please take a moment to generously write a review of this book at Amazon.com. This will only take a few minutes of your time, and you will be helping me a great deal. I sure would appreciate it.

Resources

I'd like to share with you a few resources that I believe can be very helpful in integrating Peat's views into a healthy, adaptive, flexible, and enjoyable lifestyle.

http://www.180degreehealth.com Don't be put off by the subscription nature of the site. Everything you receive through this site is free, and the founder of the site, Matt Stone, is an independent health researcher with a good heart. He manages to take the genius of Peat combined with a few others, such as Broda Barnes, and provide what turns out to be an original synthesis of these ideas combined with his experiences consulting with hundreds of people to improve their health.

http://www.youreatopia.com This site is, in my opinion, the very best resource for restrictive eating disorders that I have ever come across.

http://www.peacefulpossibility.com This is a site that I have created to share some of the stress release information that I have developed or synthesized. There are over three hours of free video training, and nothing is for sale. I am obviously biased, and everyone is different, so what works for one won't necessarily work for everyone. However, I honestly believe this is the best stress release information in the world. If that's not your cup of tea, then that's okay. I will also recommend to you HeartMath, The Work of Byron Katie, or the Sedona Method as what I believe are potentially very effective stress release techniques. Each of these can be learned through a relatively inexpensive book. (I don't recommend purchasing any of the expensive training programs, DVD programs, retreats, or other such things to learn the basics. Your investment should be <$20.)

About the Author

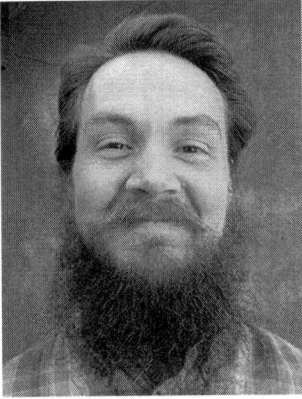

"The secret to happiness is to let go of everything - see through every assumption."

Beginning at a young age Joey Lott experienced intensifying anxiety. For several decades he lived with restrictive eating disorders, obsessions, compulsions, and an inescapable fear. By the time he was 30 years old he was physically sick, emotionally volatile, and mentally obsessed with keeping any and all unwanted thoughts and experiences at bay.

At this time Lott was living on a futon mattress in a tiny cabin in the woods. He was so sick that he could barely move. He was deeply depressed and hopeless. All this despite doing all the "right" things such as years of meditation, yoga, various "perfect" diets, clean air, and pure water.

Just when things were at their most dire, a crack appeared in the conceptual world that had formerly been mistaken for reality. By peering into this crack and underneath all the assumptions that had been unquestioned up to that moment, Lott began a great undoing. The revelation of this undoing is that reality is utterly simple, ever-present, seamless, and indivisible.

Lott's books provide a glimpse into the seamless, simple, and joyous nature of reality, offering a glimpse through the crack in conceptual worlds. Whether writing about the ultimate non-dual nature of reality, eating disorders, stress, disease, or any other subject, he offers the invitation to look at things differently, leaving behind the old, out-grown, painful limitations we have used to bind ourselves in suffering. And then, he welcomes you home to the effortless simplicity of yourself as you are.

Not sure where to begin? Pick up a copy of Lott's most popular book, *You're Trying Too Hard*, which strips away all the concepts that keep us searching for a greater, more spiritual, more peaceful life or self.

17590709R00048

Printed in Great Britain
by Amazon